I was touched by Cancer

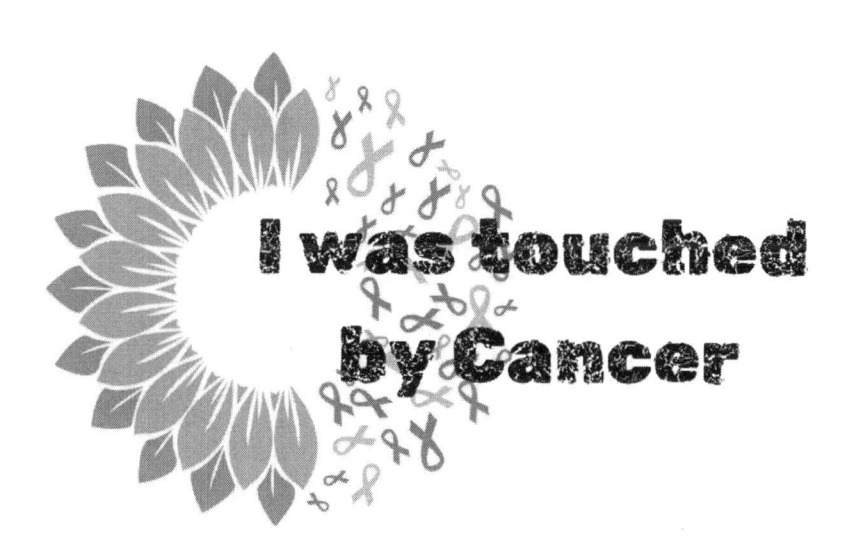

Wendy Colón Nieves

Copyright ©2024 Wendy Colón Nieves

All rights reserved.

No part of this book may be reproduced or transmitted in any form or by any means, electronic or mechanical, including photocopying, recording, or by any information storage and retrieval system, without permission in writing from the copyright owner.

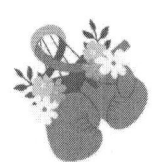

"We do not know how strong we are
until being strong is the only option
we have."

Dedication

I dedicate this small work as a posthumous tribute to those who said goodbye and who, like me, faced cancer. Those who lived similar and even more painful experiences to mine when facing this disease. To those who are now free of therapies and medications and of the poison that also spreads what still offers a few more days on this earth. To my dad, to my friend Carmen, to Milla, to Betzaida and to so many others that if I mention them, I will not finish. To those I will see again someday. For them I share my experience to raise awareness of what we can still do for friends and family members living with this disease.

Acknowledgments

I want to thank with all my heart my husband Rafael Amill and my son Nelson Gabriel Velez, both made this race less difficult. They did not let go of me even on the slopes. My husband always by my side and although sometimes silent, I know that suffering with me the uncertainty, but always presenting me in prayer to God. My son, who besides being concerned as my son, was my personal nurse, following up on everything. To both of you, thank you, a thousand thanks. It would have been more difficult without you.

I thank all the brothers in Christ who were present in one way or another: messages, songs, calls, prayers, visits, offerings, food and even cleaning. Thank you, a thousand thanks for being God's instrument to see His goodness to me.

I thank the women who have gone through the same thing and gave me advice, prayed for me and were always aware not only of how I felt physically, but also emotionally. Among them and especially Benita, a sister of the church who treats me like a daughter and Betzaida, Pastor Goveo's wife who since she knew what I was going through gave me advice and words of encouragement constantly without barely knowing me. To my friend and doctor Lucy Marrero who from the beginning was not only watching over my health but covering me with her prayers.

I thank God without a doubt because He was always by my side in this situation and calmed each of my anxieties as they arose. He certainly offered me a rest that only He could offer me amid this storm, thank you, God.

Prologue

Every book has a story behind it, a reason for being and a purpose that goes beyond its pages. This book, entitled "I was touched by cancer" is no exception. I have known Wendy Colón Nieves, the author of this book, for a little over twenty years. She has authored several books, novels, and even short stories. "Definitely Blind...", "You! Will You Help?", "Saved from What?", "God with Us", and "They Are Precious Stones Grandma!" are some of the masterful works I have had the opportunity to read.

I am privileged to call her friend and sister. Wendy is a woman with many gifts and talents, in addition to writing. We would have to write another book to list the wonderful qualities and virtues she possesses. However, what I admire most about her is her unwavering faith, and the ability she has to adapt, recover, and grow in the face of adversity, trauma, challenges, and change.

Wendy is like the Rose of Sharon, it is a flower that when detached from its stem is still alive, but the most surprising thing is that if the flower is attached again, from where it was cut, the flower comes back to life.

"I was touched by cancer" is not only a compilation of data from a testimony, but a guide to understand the transforming power of faith in the midst of adversity. It presents us with a vulnerable woman facing an unexpected and terrifying diagnosis, the uncertainty, the fear, the anguish that comes with the news and the frustration, the disappointment, and the sadness of not having the people she expected her unconditional support. She shows us how, clinging to her faith, she can pass through the valley of shadows and darkness and obtain victory, holding on to God's hand. Hallelujah!

The structure and the way it is written make it easy to read. Poems or psalms are like songs, expressing uncertainty, denial, help, hope, disappointment, peace, and faith.

This book would not have been possible without the unconditional support of her immediate family, her beloved husband Rafael Amill, who has been holding her hand at all times, her youngest son Gabriel, who honors her with his love and respect every day, and the strength that her grandchildren impart to her. And all those unsung heroes who simply became guardian angels throughout the process.

I hope that "I was touched by Cancer" will be an inspiration to write and share your own stories. To all those who have been touched by this terrible disease, may each page you read become the faith, hope and peace your soul needs.

For my part, Wendy, I thank you for being in my life and allowing me to be part of yours, my beloved Rose of Sharon.

Marilú Reyes Marzán
July 2024

"And we know that for those who love God, all things work together for good, that is, for those who are called according to his purpose." Romans 8:28 NKJV

Many times, I have read and heard this verse, but in the month of February this truth was palpable. I had pain in my left shoulder from a fall I had suffered several months before. When I went to have the MRI ordered by my doctor, I took the opportunity to have a mammogram and a Sono mammogram that I usually had in December, but after the COVID I had not continued my routine of exams.

- Your results will be ready by Friday. - the young woman who had performed the test told me.

But it was not like that, they called me the next day to inform me that my results were ready. This surprised and disturbed me, I immediately thought that the result was not good, the speed with which they performed the reading of the images and the call to tell me that I could pick them up so quickly was not normal. Even so, I went to pick them up on Thursday, when my suspicion was confirmed. The result indicated that I had a small mass in my left breast and an immediate biopsy was ordered.

This is why, even though my shoulder hurt I thanked God for the fall, because if I had not gone for the MRI I would have waited until December for my mammogram and Sono mammogram and the small mass discovered would not have been as small as the doctor indicated.

From that day on the following happened quickly. My primary care physician referred me to a breast surgeon who immediately scheduled my biopsy.

- The result will be ready in two weeks. -

Friends who knew me, understand that two weeks waiting for a result of a possible cancer was an eternity. That day, while the afternoon for many was normal, thoughts and images began to pass through my mind and I began to write about them. Amid my ordeal God was inspiring me.

At the top of the hill, uncertainty looms, to see if it can recognize the enemy crawling on the slope of the hill.
Now I understand how the psalmist was inspired by pain as well as by love. For it is that the mind runs, as if it were a girl after a butterfly that she never catches.
I do not know what awaits me ahead and despite the present threat, my sight continues to look ahead because the one who is with me is the Strong One.

And like that little girl running from side to side my mind and emotions were running. Without a clear diagnosis I did not know whether to run, cry or escape. So, in order not to torture myself and not to worry without knowing a result yet, I tried to occupy myself in everything I could so as not to give free rein to the "crazy lady of the house" as some call the mind.

The result

The biopsy result brought two interpretations that created a false hope that everything was fine. It said negative, but with atypical cells around it so surgery was recommended to remove the mass. A biopsy is a procedure that removes cells or tissue from the body, in my case, it removed a negative portion, but the story was otherwise. So, the next thing was surgery to remove it. Since I would be graduating with a master's degree in April, I begged the doctor to give me a month for the surgery so I could enjoy my accomplishment and participate in my graduation in that month. She did, but with warnings that I took the risk of it growing. This time would also allow my husband and I to raise the money to pay for the surgery.

In May I underwent a lumpectomy, which is the removal of the tumor without removing the breast. This tumor was sent for examination as the tissue removed in the biopsy.

- See you in two weeks in the office and we will see the results," the doctor told me as I was leaving the hospital after the surgery. But these two weeks were different, I felt calm, I was not anxious as when I was waiting for the biopsy results. I just took care of myself to heal as soon as possible.

Everything changes

- Well, I have the official results of what we took from you, and it is cancer. - I felt like they threw a bucket of cold water at my head, I was not expecting that news, since I had trusted the results of the biopsy.

- Do you want your husband to come in? - the nurse asked me very kindly. To which I answered:

- Yes, it is better that you explain everything to both of us. - The doctor waited for him to come in and said:

- I was telling her that the result of the mass was positive, it was a small cancerous mass. Because of this result, I have to take her to the operating room again to clean the area surrounding the mass up to two centimeters to reduce the possibility of loose cancer cells. Her cancer is ductal carcinoma in situ, so it is not one of those that spreads, so the next step after surgery will be to take radiation therapy, while the mass is sent for analysis to identify if it was caused by the hormones she was taking. -

While she was saying all this, my husband began to ask questions, he did not understand why, if the biopsy had been negative, now they were saying that I had cancer. I was trying to assimilate everything she was telling me, I was thinking about the therapies, the effects, I remembered everything my father went through when he had cancer. My eyes watered, but the doctor immediately told me:

- Your hair will not fall out; the effects are not as strong as chemotherapy. And if the mass indicates that it was due to the hormones, you will take a pill that will not give you many problems, although it is a type of oral chemo, which you would have to take for five years. -

- Well, do not say any more, let´s deal with this, operate on her, and get her therapy, we are going to get out of this," said my husband, placing his hand on mine, letting me know he was by my side.

Ductal carcinoma in situ is considered the earliest form of breast cancer. Thank God it is non-invasive, meaning it does not spread outside the breast duct and has a low risk of becoming invasive. Which brought me some peace of mind within it all.

Other problems

But when you get a diagnosis of cancer of any kind, other problems arise loud emotions and thoughts conflict with what you want. But all this is normal, some days we feel or think something and other days we see everything in a different color. Some of these emotions are anger, sadness, anguish, worry, loneliness, stress, and depression. But other days we may feel hope, new strength, and sometimes even peace.

Something that was difficult for me was to see the absence of loved ones that I thought were going to be by my side in this situation. For some reason that I did not understand and still do not understand well, they moved away and to this day have not told me anything. As if they had disappeared. I do not know if they are afraid to see me weak or if they do not know what to say, I just know they are gone, and I missed them until it did not hurt anymore. First, this affected me and that is when I wrote the following:

I see and I do not see.

How sad the nostalgia makes me when I see and do not see.
When I look around and no longer find my loved ones near me, smiling, talking or just being.
When I look back and my faded dreams of being surrounded by the bustle of the company of many.
Why does this nostalgia strike me today?
It will be the gray sky that blinds me, or the brokenness before the reality of seeing my expectations broken when the one, I love does not miss me and his voice does not reach me.
Why do we miss so much and expect so much from others knowing that they are human and therefore imperfect?
God, you are by my side, although my eyes do not see you, I feel you.
I know that by my side you cry with me, that your breath surrounds me so that I do not feel alone, even though I sometimes feel that way.
I know that I have someone who loves me, like You and other people, make me remember it, feel it, and do not doubt it. Make me see only the one who appreciates and values me, make me see only the one who loves me.
Forgive me when I go blind and do not see those, longing for others.
Forgive me when I forget that You are there, that You are enough for me not to feel alone.
Take away the gray of this sky that wants to tuck me in,
remove this cloud from my eyes so that I can admire you,
take away this sadness that wants to rule me.
Make me see the sun behind that passing cloud,
make me see your hands full of your love and kindness.
Make me see, Lord, make me see.
And while you operate on my sight, I wait confidently,
because you gave sight to the blind, and then he worshiped you.

After I wrote this, I talked to two people and told them how I felt. They made me understand that sometimes those closest to me, out of fear, denial or simply because they do not understand how necessary their company is in times like these, stay away. But if you are reading this and have a close friend or family member with cancer, do not walk away, do not leave them. It is not necessary to say much, just let them know that you are watching out for them and let them know you love them. For not doing so adds another pain to the experience of the disease. It happened to me, it hurt, but I cried and remembered that I had someone bigger than everyone who would not leave me for a moment. So, I went to Him every day and He began to let me see those who were there, those who called, those who sent me messages of encouragement, those who prayed for me. I began to realize that the body of Christ, His church was moving for me. I received messages with songs of hope, videos of Indigenous people I work with praying for my health, words of encouragement on social media and on my phone. Others brought food to my husband and me, while others came to clean my house while I recovered from my surgeries. I began to experience God's goodness through his children.

On the other hand, I was trying to manage all this roller coaster of emotions in me, and I prayed for those I saw who were affected when they knew what I was going through, some of whom surprised me when I saw them crying at the news. One of those days while I was talking to God I wrote the following:

I am not complaining, nor do I deny what I have experienced.
But I still do not know, Lord, what you want from me.
Although the announcement was not good, I was not afraid.
I do not know how to explain what I feel, I do not understand it myself.

Is it your peace, my Lord, or is it your presence with me that makes me walk in this new process?
I know that soon there will be a path that you have already traced. Is this the way you have to move me to that place? Who knows? Only you. You my guide, You, my light.

Those who are afflicted by my evil, touch them, my Lord, give them peace.
And let them see that you are with me, that you give me my strength. So that, in the midst of this, they too may know you as the Father who sustains, who does not sleep, while I sleep and who is at my side.
May he who does not understand, understand. That you sustain my soul.
May your Spirit encourage me to cross this happily.
Because by completing the test, one carat I will gain and therefore I will shine.
I will shine as you will, so that others may see in my life your character. And display the banner, that you loved me. And still do, no matter what happens.

For now, I will write, I will sing of what I feel. With my pen on a seat, waiting and writing. To give encouragement to others. I am not alone, I feel it. Feel it too, like the wind, which is not seen, but passes. What is useless snatches and what is worthwhile stands out.

Thank you, God, for what I do not yet understand, but while I understand it, make me an instrument.

The days went by and although for some people time was running, for me it stopped, it was as if it did not want to move. I was waiting for my appointment with the radiation oncologist to start my therapies, I had to wait a couple of weeks, but for me it was an eternity. While I began to internalize everything that was happening. The first months of the news I had tried to be strong, I wanted to protect my family members from the news so that they would not suffer because of me. At the end of the day, this is a mistake; our closest relatives must suffer with us to be of help, denying the reality of the disease does not help the patient at all, on the contrary, it can be detrimental.

I sought support from friends who had the same experience with this kind of cancer, this helped me a lot, it did not allow me to feel alone in the face of this disease And of course, I turned to God all the time to help me cope with the situation and the uncertainty, trying to rest in the fact that He was in control, even though I did not understand anything. In the meantime, I realized that writing down the things I was thinking and feeling was good for me, although I did not know why.

What is it about the lament, the psalm, and the song that, as you inspire me, they touch my heart?
I do not know what happens when lyrics precede pain or emotion.
I just know that something is going on in my mind and my reason, that transforms what I feel into this new expression.
Today, however, it has been the emotion that has been hammering reason.
Causing sadness in my soul and in this human heart.
Remembering the stories of so many men of God, on a day like today I can understand their mistakes and even the unwise decision, that in the face of pain and betrayal and abandonment of many they became overwhelmed, complained and some even sinned.

But writing as I do, I know that over me is your hand, keeping me from sin and complaint, though this feeling leads me to a pain that will not leave me.

God, I want to scream and cry, but that will not solve the weight I am carrying.
Only your hand God, only your grace and mercy can alleviate this sorrow. Your burden you say is light, change it for me, God change it for me, I do not want to carry mine anymore. Sitting here I wait for you and even if I can fall asleep, I know that you can come and even in my dreams penetrate and whisper in my ear that this too shall pass.
I wait for you Lord; I wait for you.
I allow no despair, for you have always come and the cloud you have dispelled. As you come and answer, and my heart bears,
I wait for you Lord; I wait for you. And my faith in you asserted.

The therapies had not yet begun, I was anxious about waiting, not knowing how much everything would cost. But immediately I began to think about how up to this day God had supplied the money for everything, at each stage of the process God went ahead and money came from somewhere. Still, I struggled daily with the thoughts that wanted to steal my peace, so when I could I wrote and wrote to seek peace.

For some unknown reason I feel like crying.
I do not know if it is I or your spirit giving me the freedom to pour myself out before you, the one who loves my soul, the one who, by kneeling down, calms me.
Today you have told me and repeated that I am not alone, and that is why I am crying, because I had not understood how close you are, I thank you Lord for everything.

*You, supplying to give me peace in the process, you calm my anxiety
when the loss of control I do not want. You show me your love in the
arms that embrace me and tell me you love me. You with me even in
dreams renewing my strength and courage. So that I do not faint,
and do not become overwhelmed no matter what happens. For you
are with me,
my refuge, my sustenance, you my friend and my encouragement.
Thank you still for what I feel, it is a sign that I am still alive and
that there is still a way to go.*

Another day of waiting and anxiety stalking me.

*Why does this anxiety haunt me when I throw it into your arms?
It managed to escape and jump into my mind and soul,
to rob me of the calm that your Spirit gives me.
The news, the uncertainty, the vanities that I see in those around me,
all try to oppress me, to sadden me. The moments of joy are so brief
and are lost in this damned anxiety, which eats away at me and
wants to overshadow them.
That is why you tell us to throw it out, to push it out of our mind and
heart, to reject it, because it has claws that poison emotion.
Lord, do not let me feel like this, abandoned in the arms of anguish
or of this dismay. Or is it that I am confusing the goal with reason?
Speak to me, God, speak to me, call my attention quickly to what you
want me to see, to where I should direct my strength.
May I not confuse the way and may I live in peace. Many times, you
have spoken to me please do it again and help me to concentrate on
what is worth Lord.
May my goal be yours; may my dream be You,
that I look neither to the right nor to the left, my Lord.
Here I await your answer, but while I do so, silence my mind Lord,
that I may not speak, that I may not cry out what is not yours my
God.*

Uncertainty became another oppressor. I was used to being in control of everything, everything was scheduled, I was highly active, and everything was on hold. But now I could not plan; I could not make decisions about what I would do tomorrow or the next week and this began to cause a void in me.

Am I in limbo? Limbo? And what is this?
A space you created, where nothing appears, there are no landscapes, no people. There are no roads, no doors. The colors do not appear, everything is of one color, it is very white, an emptiness without your voice, without your sigh, Lord.
Only an emptiness is felt, even though You fill it all.
I do not see you; I do not hear you, what is wrong with me?
It could be that I have moved away or that I have become deaf.
I know that you are calling me to peace, but I do not know how or when to enter this blank room that does not allow me to feel the peace that you offer me.
And though my feet seem steady, something happens that sways in this empty space.
You who are Lord and Master of all creation, give this room color and remove my distress. For there are many who examine my conduct in affliction, and I would like them to see in me a firm conviction that it is worthwhile to wait for you, whatever the occasion.

And they called.

    I was given an appointment, and they explained to me that first, they would do some tests and then they would determine the radiotherapy plan they were to begin with. That day that I was waiting for so long became the day when my head and my heart met, it was when the acceptance of what I was living came to my reason and understanding, which made me feel a little scared but also a little relieved. I did not have to understand anything, I was not to blame for anything, **cancer touched me**. It touched me as it can touch anyone. And now I had to move on and deal with what was left of my treatment.

They took measures here and measures there and then planned. And in your plan, Lord, did you also measure? Did you know how much I could take?
How much load I would carry without complaining, or feeling crushed?
What questions do I ask if it was you who gave man his measurements? You are balance and ruler you know well what I am made of.
You knew that today my test was difficult, that they ran out, those who were imprisoned in my eyes and I held for a while. They came out before the dark of the tube and the silence, before the fear of what follows, of the time that stops for me, while the world continues its turn.
But I am not complaining Lord, the angel that you placed there took me by the hand and told me it is okay to cry, cry, but you are going to get out of here well. This will only give you experiences to tell and to console others. So, Lord, I cry, until I can stop, and while I can I write to console others when they walk this same way. In the meantime, renew my strength to go on as you have done so many times in the face of this same feeling.

Finally, my radiation therapies began. Radiation therapy is a treatment where the cancer area is bombarded with high doses of radiation to destroy or slow the growth of cancer cells. Radiation therapy does not immediately destroy these cells. It takes many days for them to die, and they continue to die even weeks after the end of radiation therapy. In my case, I would have thirty-five therapies in a machine that moved and sent the radiation from many directions and the last of them would treat the specific area where the mass was removed.

In my case, as in the case of many, the experience with the machine is not the most pleasant thing we go through. First, we arrived with fear, uncertain of what it would be like, will it hurt, what will it feel like, and how long will I be in it. But the answers came immediately. It didn't hurt, but in the end, I felt very hot in the treated area. It only took fifteen minutes each session from Monday to Friday. But even though it did not hurt, and it was fast, I did not like the machine. I came out of there feeling as tired as if I had run a ten-kilometer marathon. So, from there to rest, I could not do more, it was as if the machine exhausted my energy with the cells it burned.

That machine that burns.

You pushed me with violence, into a machine that burns. But He will help me, He who breathes and gives life, protects me from that evil. His size impresses me, that noise is even frightening because it deceives, and although what it does kills and burns, my soul cannot touch, like the one who always pursues me and wants to put me in chains. Christ comes to my rescue; He has put Himself in my place. I am shot and He burns, He hurts and not me. I cry only when I think that He, himself climbed for me to this table that is my cross, but also my hope, that there remains what tries to leave me in darkness. I am passing this Calvary, I know that soon I will hear; that you are free, it is finished, I paid for you. Thank you, God, you have not left me. You have walked beside me and when I have been very weak, you have carried me in your arms. Thank you, my beloved Lord, I praise you, my God, I praise you.

Day 19

Today I am tired, and cloudy as the day. I feel my goal is far away. More than the damage to my skin, it is my being that is beaten. My mood has weakened, today I cannot smell the flowers or hear the birds, they are also silent with me. There are only sixteen more to go, but they are uphill, that is why I see that my feet go slower every day. Fatigue is with me walking now and although You and many support me, I feel sad Lord. Touch my soul my God, my spirit, and my emotion, do not let me give up, give me a touch, new strength, give me one last push to reach the top, and sing a song. Tell others you can, even if it hurts, even if it tires, even if you want to take it off, look up, keep walking that, like me, you will get there. As I came to sing to them, give me your hand Lord, hold me in this moment, do not let go, please.

Something very difficult, while you are in radiation therapy, is that it reminds you daily that you are facing a disease that is a constant threat. A threat to our lives, our emotional health, our minds, and even to our family who suffer with us because they love us. And although one knows that treatment is part of recovery, there are times when it does not calm the feelings and thoughts. Tough times come, even if we have faith, but it is okay, when we express our feelings to God He will surely understand and comfort us when necessary.

What Anger

Today I feel terribly upset, what anger, Lord.
Today they stop everything I know with good reason.
But I cannot avoid this anger, my God.
It is not with you that I am angry, it is not with anyone, Lord.
These are the marks that this evil insists on leaving on my body without mercy.
But the astute doctor said enough, is enough, you have to stop, you have to give time to time so you can heal. But even though I knew it was a wise decision, anger took over my mind and heart. What anger do I feel for not being in control of time, of my future, but who is in control, Lord?

If you have already numbered my days, my God, why this anger I feel when I should rest? Stop me is your command and because I am rebellious. Though angry I feel forgive me, my God, and take away this anger that has me out of control. I need more patience and a little more of your peace to endure the waiting and learn to enjoy it. Forgive me, Lord, and do not let this anger grow anymore, in the meantime, while you are at it, take away the anxiety as well. That which enters my mind at times to disturb, putting also sadness thus robbing me of your peace. Help me to discard it, to tear it away and rest. That is what you want and that is what I want to learn, to rest. Here I wait for your help, your voice I want to hear you tell me: "Receive it, daughter, receive it, receive my peace now."

In my opinion, the stages of grief are also stages that we experience in the face of an illness over which we have no control, so I reached the stage of anger, a mixture of sadness and frustration for not being able to change my situation and having to let someone else be in charge of my diary and against whom we are also unjustly angry. But like all anger passes, and even more so if we turn to God to help us deal with it by accepting that whatever happens is still under His control.

But waiting is desperate and to be honest I was desperate not knowing when I would resume the therapies, much less when I would finish them. As the days passed the fight in my mind was constant with negative thoughts that the enemy fires using as ammunition the information of thousands of cancer cases. But one day I began to remember the times I have been able to die, the times God spared me from death because it was not my time to go to his presence in heaven. I began to imagine how God has sent angels to watch over us, to fight fights we do not even see and to watch over our steps. And that day I wrote the following:

Angels

I was thinking my God, I was thinking of your army Lord.
How many angels of heaven are at our side, O God?
In your Word I see them caring for yours with words of encouragement,
with food and water as well.
You protect them, you defend them from the attacking enemy.
But I see that they still walk around us.
Your little ones are also taking care of us today.
They encourage us, hug us, and even make us laugh,
to ease our burden and take away our pain.
They protect us with swords and with hugs as well.
They guard us from the enemy that prowls all around us.
But also, the one that enters our mind to lurk.
I have seen them remarkably close; they have left traces of their presence at my side.
They have taken care of me, they have freed me when I sleep, and when I travel.
And now there are three who, although in disguise,
I know you sent them.
I am lifted from a table where they burn any cell that wants to torture me.
But there they also cheer me up and make me smile, one sings or tries to, another tries to paint, and another with her cold hands reminds me that I am alive, but her sweet words don't move, I move you, remind me every day of your care my Lord.
They do not know that I know that you sent them, that they were chosen for this mission with me. God bless them, be with them, continue to use them, Lord, giving peace, and encouragement to those who arrive there. To that room that is cold, where one enters with fear, but where they touch us with your hand, with your love.
Thank you, Lord, for them, a thousand thanks, my God.

Many things are experienced when one is going through cancer and its treatment: sadness, anxiety, loneliness, fear, anger, and others. And it is not easy to express how we feel, sometimes we want to shut ourselves away and not talk to anyone, others want to shout to everyone how we feel, but in the end, the best thing to do is to talk to God. He and only He can offer us what we need for any feeling we have and many times through the people we least imagine. I wish more people would be sensitive to God's voice and use their hands and mouths to encourage and embrace those going through these experiences of pain and treatment.

The Way

On my way to my last therapy, my chest tightened, but not from radiation, but from emotion.
The excitement of closing this detour on my way.
A mixture of emotion and thoughts. Joy mixed with gratitude but that made me cry. Crying at the thought of how God has accompanied me, how He has never left me. A sorrow if I am left to think of those beside me who sit without knowing you, Lord,
without feeling your great love that can comfort them in this challenging time.
I pray for them my God, that they may meet you and experience your care, my Lord. Today I am thankful for so much my God, my husband, and my son, none of them left me alone.

They have been here by my side even without knowing what to do for me, but their very presence gave me strength and encouragement along the way. Although they never understood why you let me go through this ordeal, I only know that they were asking you to give me new strength and never leave me.

What a mixture of feelings when I left that place because, although a chapter was closed there, I will have to turn daily to your mercy, Lord, because uncertainty will always be a threat to my mind and my heart as well. But I know that you understand me, my Lord, that it is not faith that I lack, it is the defect of my race that daily thinks, and doubts, instead of coming to you daily to receive the necessary measure of faith that I need to survive. Thank you, God, my God thank you, for this opportunity to continue walking and to continue illuminating with your oil my Lord.

What is next?

After cancer, nothing is the same. Not only your routine and your pace but also your way of seeing everything. Everything has another color, another value. You appreciate more the things that surround us, and that God gives us every day, like the breeze and the smell of rain. We value the time we spend with our loved ones, even if they are not perfect. We avoid toxic people and sad news so as not to get sick again. You live more slowly but more deeply.

But the care does not stop. More doctors are visited, and treatments are continued that bring with them side effects that become daily struggles. A preventive follow-up program is maintained, in short, everything changes. You hear the expression remission, that the cancer is gone, and/or that the suspicious cells are disappearing. I thought I would hear you are cancer-free from the mouth of one of the doctors, but I think they do not say it so that you do not get careless and follow the next treatment. Anyway, the struggles with emotions continue, one day you are happy and full of joy because you survived the experience, and another day you fear it will come back. Sometimes you resent the losses, you have to accept the new reality, the new appearance, and forgive those who were not there. In the face of this, you have to remember that you are not alone, many women go through this and are also still struggling. We must celebrate when joy appears, when the breeze caresses us and we enjoy the company of someone dear to us, celebrating the opportunity to feel without fear and experience that momentary joy.

My God will supply...

I want to add to these letters, that God not only accompanied me and showed Himself through many who in one way or another were by my side, but He, who allowed me to live this experience, took care of paying all the expenses of my treatment. So, I want to share with you the testimony of how He supplied everything.

As many of you know, healthcare costs have increased terribly and in the case of everything related to cancer, it is even more expensive. Although I have a medical plan, it only covers portions of the treatments, and the rest I must pay for myself, with what they call a deductible, which varies depending on the treatment. But God, who knows that I only depend on a small pension, stepped in and began to make up for it. As I do not want to lose any detail, I will write this enumerating the moments in which God's wallet opened to give the money that his daughter needed.

1. Biopsy- When I saw the breast surgeon for the biopsy, I was told that I needed approval of my treatment plan, so I was scheduled for the following week for the biopsy. The cost to me, after the plan contribution, would be $380.00 which on the day I saw the surgeon I did not have. But four days before the biopsy I received money back from my credit card, and how much did I receive? $680.00, of which $300.00 to fix my car that I had left on the road that same day and $380.00 for my biopsy.

2.	Second operation - on May 23 I had undergone surgery and with the savings we had and some things I sold we completed the deductible for this operation. But I had to have another one on June 23 and for that one we had nothing. But as soon as I knew I was going to have another surgery, I prayed and told God one morning, *"You are allowing another surgery, you have to pay for it, we don't have anything."* That same afternoon I got a call from the church, and they said, *"Don't worry about your surgery, we are going to pay for it."* I could only look up and thank God for hearing me and responding so quickly.

3.	Study (MRI)- As part of some studies I had to have an MRI but the last time they tried it was a nightmare. I suffer from claustrophobia which does not allow me to calmly enter the famous tube of that machine. So, I looked for a place that had the machine open, but this cost me $100.00 which we did not have. I told my husband: *well, let us wait to get paid and take out the $100.00 that we use to buy food because I cannot enter the tube.* And so, we did. But when I was waiting for them to call me to pay, I heard a ting! On my cell phone, some brothers from the church were sending me an offering of $100.00. Once again God paid.

4.   Radiation therapy- My husband remembered that he had a cancer policy and thought it covered me as well because I was his spouse. Indeed, it did. This policy works on a reimbursement basis for some expenses. So, we called, and I got my bearings and submitted all the paperwork for what I had already done. They sent me a percentage of what I had already spent, and I kept it to use to pay for the radiation therapy. I imagined that this was extremely expensive, but I did not know how much, but God did. While I was waiting for the approval of the medical plan for my treatment and to know how much they would cover and how much I would have to pay, God worked. I began to receive many offerings, money came not only from people in Puerto Rico but also from El Salvador, Argentina, the United States, and Spain. Curious, I looked in the bank account, and between the reimbursements and the offerings I already had $3,500.00. I told my husband: *"If God is sending this money, it is because these therapies will be very expensive, so let's see how we will pay for everything"*. That same day I got a call from the therapies office and the girl said, *"Hello, I am calling to tell you that the medical plan approved your therapies. The cost of your therapies is $17,250.00 but you will only have to pay 20% which is $3,450.00."* As I was speechless, the girl tells me, *"I know it is a lot of money, but don't worry, when you come to the office, we will work out a payment plan for you."* That is when without getting out of my astonishment I told her, *"I'm not speechless because of that, but because my dad knew how much it was and gave me the money before you called me, but when I go to the office, I'll tell you everything."* So, I paid my $3,450 and the rest ($50.00) was used to pay for parking every time I went to my therapy. ;)

I share this last point because we must recognize that God is our everything. That we have a father who knows what we need. That God also meddles in our finances and that our wallets are His wallets, for the money is His. So, He knows what we need, and He will supply what we need.

Final words

You may wonder why I authored this little book, for what? First for me and second for you. For me because it is my way of sharing my experience with other people so that they know or remember that they are not alone. Many of us will be going through sickness or hardship, but there is still hope, not only for today but also for tomorrow. That, if we are healed well, it is ok and if we are not healed is ok also because we will see God's gracious hand in our situation. For you, who have not gone through something similar, I write so that you understand the sick person, even the one who trusts in God, who is human and doubts, fears, and cries. Do not leave him alone, you do not have to be there all the time, just long enough for him to know that he can count on you. You do not know what to say? You do not have to say anything, just be by his side and hold his hand, he will understand what you want to say.

So, I hope that this little book will be an inspiration to the sick, to wait on God and trust that He is at their side. And to others to let God use them. Be his hands to embrace and his mouth to comfort and express love and empathy.

"And we know that for those who love God, all things work together for good, that is, for those who are called according to His purpose."
Romans 8:28 KJV

Made in the USA
Middletown, DE
15 October 2024